Flaxseed Oil

Rich Source of Beneficial Omega-3s

Second Edition
Revised and Updated

Kate Udall

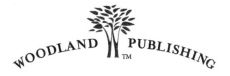

Copyright © 2007 Kate Udall

All rights reserved. No part of this publication may be reproduced, stored in a retrieval system, or transmitted in any form without the prior written permission of the copyright owner.

For ordering information and bulk order discounts, contact:
Woodland Publishing, 448 East 800 North, Orem, UT 84097
Toll-free telephone: (800) 777-BOOK

Please visit our Web site: www.woodlandpublishing.com

Note: The information in this book is for educational purposes only and is not recommended as a means of diagnosing or treating an illness. All matters concerning physical and mental health should be supervised by a health practitioner knowledgeable in treating that particular condition. Neither the publisher nor the author directly or indirectly dispenses medical advice, nor do they prescribe any remedies or assume any responsibility for those who choose to treat themselves.

A cataloging-in-publication record for this book is available from the Library of Congress.

ISBN: 978-1-58054-438-2

Printed in the United States of America

Contents

Introduction 5

Essential Fatty Acids: A Definition 6

Fish vs. Flaxseed 7

Negative Effects of Fatty-Acid Imbalance 7

The Value of Supplementing with Flaxseed Oil 8

Functions of Essential Fatty Acids 9

Health Benefits of a Balanced Fatty-Acid Intake 10

Flax and Lignans 16

Flax and Fiber 17

Selecting a Source 17

Additional Roles of Flaxseed 19

Recent Research 19

Conclusion 20

References 21

Introduction

Most Americans are aware of the connection between a high-fat diet and serious health problems such as heart disease, high cholesterol, diabetes, and cancer. But what many people may not know is that the kind of fat we take into our bodies is as important as the amount. This notion, first observed by researchers in the early 1950s, is made particularly clear by a comparison of the Eskimo diet and the standard American diet (SAD). Eskimos routinely eat a diet high in animal fat but do not suffer from cardiovascular disease as Americans do.

The explanation for this phenomenon is that the Eskimos eat a great deal of fish, a food high in unsaturated fats, which help to limit the harmful effects of saturated fats. If we look at this in a somewhat simplified way, we could say that the relationship between the two types of fat is that they work to cancel each other out. While saturated fats—those found in margarine, shortening, and most prepared foods—actually negatively affect the way the body uses unsaturated fats, the reverse is also true. A diet that includes low levels of saturated fats and high levels of unsaturated ones can actually work to protect the body against heart disease and cancer.

This counteractive effect works because of the presence of two essential fatty acids, or EFAs. These fatty acids are called essential because the body needs them for proper function but cannot produce them on its own. Dr. Joyce Nettleton refers to them as "absolutely essential" because without them deficiency symptoms develop and growth ceases. Since the body can't synthesize EFAs to form other fatty acids, it relies on food sources to supply them ready-made. Problems result from the fact that the typical American diet does not include a sufficient amount of EFAs.

Essential Fatty Acids: A Definition

Much research and attention has focused on two primary types of EFAs that include two polyunsaturated fats—linoleic and alpha linolenic acids. The body needs both of these acids to function properly, and they are necessary for normal cell structure. The basic difference between the two is in their molecular structure Dr. Michael T. Murray, ND, explains: "Although both linoleic acid and alpha-linolenic acid are eighteen-carbon-length fatty acids, alpha-linolenic acid has three unsaturated bonds while linoleic acid has only two. The location of the first unsaturated bond is different as well. Alpha-linolenic acid's first unsaturated bond occurs at the third carbon, hence its classification as omega-3 oil. Linoleic acid's first unsaturated bond is at the sixth carbon; it is an omega-6 oil."

From Murray's explanation, two oils are identified: omega-3 and omega-6. The body needs a balance of the two fatty-acids to function at an optimal level. Linoleic acid is an omega-6 fatty acid and alpha-linoleic acid is an omega-3 fatty-acid.

These fatty acids have distinct properties and functions. Linoleic acid has been shown in numerous studies to be responsible for the transport of water across the skin and the proper functioning of the pituitary gland. These functions make linoleic acid beneficial in the treatment of many skin conditions and a likely tool in successful growth and development therapies.

Alpha-linolenic acid has important functions as well. Recent research has established that it offers protective effects against both coronary heart disease and stroke. Among other things, alpha-linolenic acid is also the precursor to two types of necessary omega-3 fatty acids, eicosapentaenoic acid (EPA) and docosahexaenoic acid (DHA). That is, alpha-linolenic acid helps the body create the other two types. These omega-3 acids combine to benefit those suffering from migraines, arthritis, and high cholesterol levels.

Much has been written about the value of foods that are high in omega-3 fatty acids. Fish oil (marine lipids) and flaxseed oil have been identified as two rich sources of omega-3 fatty acids. Fish oil is an established source of omega-3 fatty acids. There is much conclusive research to back up its reputation as a cardiovascular disease–fighting agent. Generally, however, most Americans do not eat enough cold-water fish to adequately provide the necessary amount of omega-3 fatty acids.

The second source of omega-3s is flaxseed oil. Studies have shown that flaxseed oil offers many benefits in fighting disease and improving overall health. But should you choose fish oil or flaxseed oil? Nutrition experts have some interesting things to say about the benefits of flaxseed over fish oils.

Fish vs. Flaxseed

Hundreds of detailed scientific studies have shown that supplementation with fish oils offers beneficial health effects, especially in improving cardiovascular function, including lowering cholesterol levels and blood pressure. Fish oils are composed of two fatty acids, EPA and DHA, which can be manufactured in the human body from alpha-linolenic acid, the chief fatty acid found in flaxseed oil.

Flaxseed oil may be a better choice when you consider that many fish oil supplements have been shown to be contaminated with toxic derivatives known as lipid peroxides. While extra vitamins and other antioxidant nutrients offer some protection against these compounds, avoiding the intake of lipid peroxides is safer. Advantages of flaxseed oil over fish oil also include:

- Taste and smell is more pleasant—no more fish burps!
- Higher omega-3 concentration
- Lower processing costs
- Less prone to rancidity
- Not contaminated with chemicals and heavy metals

Negative Effects of Fatty-Acid Imbalance

The standard American diet is especially deficient in omega-3 fats, whose primary source is alpha-linolenic acid. The negative effects of this deficiency are numerous. Most nutrition experts believe the optimum ratio of omega-6 to omega-3 oils is between 3:1 and 4:1. But the estimate of the ratio in the diet of most Americans is 20:1—the level of omega-6 is twenty times that of omega-3 oil.

Clearly, such an imbalance is not conducive to good health. Maintaining a better ratio by increasing the intake of omega-3 fatty acids can noticeably improve body functions. As Dr. William E. Connor notes: "It is probable ... that there has always been the proper balance between these two groups of essential fatty acids, but in the modern era with the provision of inexpensive vegetable oils, it is possible that the pendulum for increased dietary omega-6 fatty acids in the form of linoleic acid has swung too far and the intake of omega-3 acids has actually declined."

Omega-3 deficiency has resulted in many negative effects in our health and lifestyle. Some signs of EFA deficiency in the diet include skin dryness, goose flesh on the backs of the arms, loss of hair, and changes in immune function such as an increased susceptibility to infection. In fact, a study done as early as 1929 demonstrated the essential quality of linolenic acid. Those researchers documented the symptoms of EFA deficiency as scaly skin, below-normal growth rate, excess water through the skin, kidney malfunction, fatty liver, poor reproductive performance, and reduced life span.

Because omega-6 fats are usually found to such a higher degree in most American diets, we probably need to focus more on finding better sources of omega-3s. Omega-3 fats are found in walnuts, winter wheat, and soy oil. They can also be found in cold water fish, such as mackerel, salmon, herring, tuna, and sardines.

The Value of Supplementing with Flaxseed Oil

As discussed previously, because typical Western diets are deficient in omega-3 fatty acids, flaxseed oil is very useful in helping to even out the ratio between omega-3 and omega-6 fatty acids for a healthier balance. While other plant seeds—corn, sunflowers, and peanuts—contain omega-6 fatty acids, flaxseed alone contains such a large amount of the essential omega-3 fatty acids.

Flax, a blue flowering crop grown for its oil-rich seeds, has been harvested and used in the diet since ancient times. Around 3000 BC Baby-

Ionians are recorded to have used it. And in 650 BC, Hippocrates wrote about using flax for the relief of abdominal pain. In the eighteenth century, Charlemagne considered flax so important for the health of his subjects that he passed laws and regulations regarding its consumption. Even though early peoples may not have known exactly what natural properties in flax made it such a valuable part of their diet, they recognized the flax as a useful plant.

Today, we are once again recognizing the value of flaxseed oil. Although much research is still in progress to determine all of the health benefits of flax, we now recognize that a large part of its nutritional value comes from its natural oil content. Flaxseed is about 41 percent oil, but very little of that is saturated. More than 70 percent of the fat in flaxseed oil is the healthful polyunsaturated type. In fact a unique feature of flaxseed is the high ratio of alpha-linolenic acid (omega-3) to linoleic acid (omega-6).

Functions of Essential Fatty Acids

The linoleic and alpha-linolenic acids found in flax are necessary for two reasons. First, they are responsible for forming a group of hormone-like compounds called prostaglandins. These are made in every single cell in the body. Their function is to regulate cell activities. The effects of prostaglandin production, for which omega-3 oils are responsible, include many disease-fighting benefits. They play a role in the performance in the cardiovascular, reproductive, immune, and central nervous systems.

Body tissue synthesizes prostaglandins and creates a balance between two different types of prostaglandins that initiate opposite responses. A fatty-acid deficiency could disrupt this balance, setting into motion undesirable and often-harmful physical effects.

The second reason that essential fatty acids are essential is that they are vital to the cell membrane structure. They make them impermeable. The permeability of the membrane helps in the protection of cells against invading bacteria, toxins, infection, and viruses. The cell membrane also facilitates the flow of nutrients and waste material in and out of the cell. It is easy to see that the human body must rely on adequate dietary supplies of linoleic and alpha-linolenic acids to function normally. Supplementation through flaxseed oil is the most convenient and nutritionally sound way to do this.

Health Benefits of a Balanced Fatty-acid Intake

Obviously, a balance in essential fatty acids is necessary for many body functions. It also promotes good overall health. In particular, the omega-3 fatty acids are essential for human development and important in achieving good health throughout life. The tissues of the body require the omega-3 and omega-6 fatty acids for proper functioning. Supplementing your diet with omega-3 oils can help to prevent and sometimes treat:

- High cholesterol levels
- Strokes
- Cancer
- Psoriasis and eczema
- Heart disease
- High blood pressure
- Multiple sclerosis
- Rheumatoid arthritis

The following overview discusses in more detail the individual conditions mentioned above that can be improved by omega-3 supplementation through flaxseed oil.

High Cholesterol

Diets high in fat, particularly saturated fat, are linked with high blood-cholesterol levels, a risk factor for cardiovascular diseases such as coronary heart disease (CHD) and stroke. Diet therapies to reduce build-up of cholesterol and risk of CHD often focus mainly on reducing total and saturated fat intake. Dietary interventions that reduce saturated fat intake level by just 3 percent could prevent about 100,000 new cases of CHD by the year 2005.

When dietary saturated fats are decreased, they can be replaced with polyunsaturated fats, including the omega-3 fatty acids that lower both total cholesterol and LDL-cholesterol. A the precursor to EPA and DHA—the EFAs that lower cholesterol levels—alpha-linolenic acid is a highly essential acid in the diet of those wishing to reduce cholesterol levels or maintain healthy levels. These long-chain omega-3 fatty acids have been shown to reduce blood triglycerides, increase blood HDL cholesterol (the "good" cholesterol), reduce blood pressure, reduce platelet activity, and reduce neutrophil activity—all actions that help lower the risk of CDH. Again, flaxseed is a very rich source of this fatty acid, and the only rich plant source.

The alpha-linolenic acid found in flax influences physiological processes and disease risk. In clinical trials, alpha-linolenic acid exerts positive effects on blood lipids, the potentially harmful fats found in the blood. One study found that alpha-linolenic acid was effective in lowering total plasma cholesterol in eight healthy men, aged twenty to thirty-four years. Further, in fifteen men and women, the addition of fifteen grams of milled flaxseed to their diet produced significant reductions in total cholesterol levels. Blood triglycerides decreased slightly, but not significantly. These findings suggest that modest reductions in total cholesterol can be achieved by adding flaxseed to the diet. Substituting alpha-linolenic acid (so abundant in flaxseed oil) for saturated fats enhances these beneficial effects.

Heart Disease

A person's genetic inheritance influences the likelihood of premature heart disease, but it is becoming increasingly clear that modifying one's lifestyle can do much to improve upon the effects of one's genes. Heart disease, mainly heart attacks, account for nearly one of every three deaths in the united states, about six million a year. Although the annual rate of death from heart disease has been declining since the late 1960s, it remains the leading cause of death in the United States and a major cause in other Western countries.

The good news is that people can reduce their risk of developing and dying from heart disease, as well as lower the likelihood of having a premature heart attack. The most important strategy for an individual who wishes to avoid heart disease is to adopt prevention habits. Some of the most crucial prevention tactics are:

1. Avoid smoking.
2. Maintain a desirable blood cholesterol level.
3. Keep blood pressure in the normal range.
4. Regularly engage in aerobic exercise.

Besides these lifestyle habits, certain substances and nutrients have been shown to reduce the risk of heart disease. Alpha-linolenic acid is one such substance that can be taken as supplementation to improve the body's ability to fight heart disease. The exact mechanism by which alpha-linolenic acid protects against stroke and myocardial infarction, arrhythmia, and other cardiovascular events is not known, but one way in which alpha-linolenic acid can help can lower heart disease risk is by modifying membrane phospholipids. A recent study suggests that the alpha-linolenic content of blood phospholipids and triglycerides can be increased two- to eight-fold by supplementing the diet with flaxseed or flaxseed oil for a period of four weeks. Increasing the omega-3 fatty acid content of membrane phospholipids increases membrane fluidity and alters membrane function, which "may reduce cardiovascular disease risk by influencing calcium ion exchange across the membrane."

The study of how alpha-linolenic acid protects against cardiovascular disease is still new. Future research will likely clarify its physiological effects and its benefits in reducing the risk of cardiovascular diseases.

Strokes

Stroke has two main causes: the clogging of an artery from atherosclerosis, a condition in which the vessel walls thicken and plaque builds up on the arteries; or hemorrhaging caused by a break in the artery. Stroke is the third leading cause of death in the United States, after heart disease and cancer.

Alpha-linolenic acid may lower the risk of stroke, according to data from the Multiple Risk Factor Intervention Trial (MRFIT). An analysis of MRFIT subjects with stoke incidents who were followed for six to nine years found that the alpha-linolenic content of blood cholesterol esters and phospholipids was inversely associate with risk of stroke. Each increase in alpha-linolenic acid was associated with a 30 percent reduction in stroke risk.

High Blood Pressure

Differences in blood pressure among populations have been known for decades, but causes of the variation are less certain. Are they genetic, dietary, stress-related, or environmental? Certain genetic susceptibility to hypertension has been ascribed to American blacks, and familial predisposition to high blood pressure is well known.

There appears to be no single cause of hypertension, but several of the body's systems are involved, including the endocrine, cardiovascular, and nervous systems. External factors including obesity, alcohol intake, stress, and consumption of sodium, potassium, calcium, dietary fat, and certain fatty acids, make susceptible individual—millions of us—develop the condition sooner or later. The major risk to health from high blood pressure is stroke, the third most frequent cause of death in many industrial countries and a leading cause of disability. In the early 1980s, several studies suggested that omega-3 fatty acids lowered blood pressure by small but statistically significant amounts. Healthy males consumed fish oils or fatty fish and experienced a reduction in blood pressure. Alpha-linolenic acid has also been suggested as a likely factor in lower levels of hypertension.

Rheumatoid Arthritis

Although rheumatoid arthritis has probably been around for centuries, its cause remains a mystery. Most researchers agree that autoimmunity is involved in the progression of arthritis, but the primary cause of the disease is less certain. Its debilitating effects, however, are familiar to some forty million people in the United States. It is estimated that about one percent of the population worldwide is afflicted with the disease, yet mortality from arthritis is likely underestimated. Unfortunately, arthritis has frequently dietary benefits tend to be greeted with skepticism, if not completely ignored.

The effectiveness of EFAs in helping rheumatoid arthritis has been validated through modern science. Scientists at the University of Pennsylvania conducted research on the effects of alpha-linolenic acid on arthritis sufferers. Six out of seven patients receiving doses of alpha-linolenic acid experienced reduced inflammation of the synovial fluid in the joints.

In a later twenty-four week trial study, fourteen rheumatoid arthritis patients took doses of linolenic acid and the "number of tender joints" decreased by 36 percent. The "degree of tenderness" decreased by 45 percent, and the "stiffness of joints upon arising" diminished by 33 percent. Those patients receiving placebos, on the other hand, experienced no change.

Multiple Sclerosis

Multiple sclerosis (MS) is a disease of the central nervous system that destroys the myelin sheaths that cover each nerve, creating inflammation. Symptoms include blurred vision, dizziness, numbness, weakness, tremors, slurred speech, and staggering. The underlying cause of the disease is unknown, as is a cure. But we do know that stress and poor nutrition may contribute to its progression. MS usually occurs in individuals between the ages of twenty-five and forty. It often goes into remission for periods of time only to reappear.

In the 1950's Roy Swank was the first to propose a link between fat, particularly saturated fatty acids, and MS. Hugh Sinclair (1956) amplified this hypothesis in a provocative letter to the editor of Lancet. Sinclair warned about the "development of relative fatty acid deficiency," by which term he meant the diminishing proportion of essential fatty acids in the diet owing to the increased consumption of animal fats and the removal of vegetable oils in food processing. Associated with such a deficiency, he contended, was the development of "a deficiency of normal phospholipids (or presence of abnormal phospholipids) in the nervous system causing defective structure including demyelination." Since that time, many studies have born out his conclusion.

Current research is investigating the possibility that multiple sclerosis is at least partially caused by prostaglandin deficiency. Prostaglandins, as mentioned earlier, are created from EFAs. Because some MS patients have reduced levels of alpha-linolenic acid, it is likely that flaxseed oil supplementation would be beneficial.

Psoriasis

Psoriasis is a skin disease characterized by patches of scaly skin, most commonly on the knees, elbows and scalp, but possibly anywhere on the body. Symptoms often flare up and then go into remission, and arthritis may be present. It is considered essentially incurable by conventional methods have offered considerable hope. Treatment with steroids is common, but steroids have offered no real cure.

It is known that an essential fatty acid deficiency in humans results in skin rashes that resemble eczema and psoriasis. Flaxseed oil is among the natural therapeutic agents for psoriasis because of its rich EFA content. Some psoriasis sufferers also see improvements by eliminating the harmful dietary fats found in such sources as fried foods, margarine, and hydrogenated oils, because such fats interfere with EFA metabolism.

In 1986, Ziboh, et al., showed that the dietary supplementation of psoriasis patients with omega-3 oil for eight weeks was accompanied by mild to moderate improvement in psoriatic lesions in eight out of thirteen patients. Two patients reported significant alleviation of their symptoms. Other subsequent studies have shown the same conclusions.

Cancer

Most of us are aware that certain types of fats have been linked with the development of malignancies, and there is some evidence that obtaining a consistent supply of omega-3 oils may help to prevent these fat-sensitive types of cancer. In addition, cancers such as breast, colon, prostate, and omega-3 oils. One of the most fascinating properties of this oil is its ability to neutralize the undesirable effects of other fatty acids found in certain vegetables and meats.

It is precisely for this reason that supplementation with a flax source is so vital. Studies at Cornell University concluded that the omega-3 fatty acids fond in flax have great potential to inhibit the development of certain cancer: "While breast tumors in experimental animals differ in important ways from those in women, laboratory studies of dietary fat have clearly shed light upon the factors affecting the relationship of fat consumption and human breast cancer risk. . . . Research scientists have also discovered that different types of fat vary in their ability to promote the growth of animal tumors. . . . The safest were the omega-3 unsaturated oils."

Flax and Lignans

While it is important to stress that the fatty acids found in flax are essential, research also suggests that flax contains substances called lignans, special compounds that demonstrate some impressive health benefits. Lignans seem to be responsible for aiding the immune system in various ways as well as helping to prevent some types of cancers. The lignan component of flax makes it even a more beneficial form of supplementation.

Flax is one of the richest sources of lignans, which are compounds that can interfere with estrogen metabolism in animals and humans. It is this that gives lignans the capability to help in the prevention of fat- and hormone-sensitive types of cancer.

Population studies of diet and disease risk suggest and anti-cancer for lignans and other phytoestrogens. Populations with high intakes of phytoestrogens—such as high-fiber diet rich in lignans from vegetables and grains—have lower incidence and mortality rates of breast, endometrial, and prostate cancers. These studies are suggestive but not conclusive. Long-term studies of flaxseed effects in women with breast cancer are underway.

The benefits of lignans also include positive effects in antibacterial, antifungal, and antiviral activity which help the immune system function at optimal capacity.

Lignans from pine cones have been shown to inhibit replication of the human immunodeficiency virus. The implications of these findings and other potential health benefits of lignans are still being investigated, but there is no doubt that lignans can boost the body's ability to fight virus and infection.

Flax and Fiber

Although research is still underway to learn all of the health benefits of flax, it has been established that flax besides containing essential fatty acids and lignans, is a good source of fiber. Several studies confirm that flaxseed can be a cholesterol-lowering agent just like oat bran, fruit pectin, and other food ingredients that contain soluble fiber. By packaging both omega-3 fatty acids and soluble fiber together, flaxseed presents two ingredients that favor healthy blood lipid patterns. The nutrient make-up of flax is given below.

Nutrient Profile of Flax per 100 grams/3oz.

Food Energy	450 calories
Fat	41 grams
Total Dietary Fiber	28 grams
Protein	20 grams

Analyzed by the American Oil Chemists' Society, which is based on the Federation of Oils, Seeds and Fats Association Ltd. official method.

Flaxseed contains healthy amounts of both soluble and insoluble fiber. Scientists at the American National Caner Institute singled out flaxseed as one of six foods that deserved special study. The reason: flaxseed, as has been discussed, showed potential cancer-fighting ability.

The structural components of flaxseed—high amounts of omega-3 fatty acids, lignans, and soluble and insoluble fiber—make it a necessary and beneficial source of supplementation in the diet

Selecting a Source

An important consideration when selecting a healthy diet is in choosing sources of EFAs. Because EFAs are fragile and are easily damaged by air, high temperatures, and food processing, even if you are careful to use vegetable oils for cooking, you likely aren't getting the EFAs you need. Unfortunately, most of the oil we consume today has been heaIily processed, damaging the EFAs. Choosing a flax oil will present the same considerations: you'll want to choose a flaxseed oil that has not been damaged by processing.

Not all flax oils are created equal. There is tremendous variation in quality and purity as a result in differences in how the oil is expressed. Most flaxseed oils are produced by mechanically pressing out the oil through an expeller. During this process a tremendous amount of pressure and heat can be generated. The higher the heat, the better the yield of oil. Temperatures generally reach 200 degrees F. interestingly, flax oil processed in this manner can still be referred to as cold-pressed because no external source of heat is added.

Although high temperatures will provide a greater quantity of oil, they produce a lower quality oil. Many manufacturers will sacrifice quality for quantity. However, consumers must be aware that because flax oil is a highly unsaturated oil, it is extremely susceptible to damage by heat, light, and oxygen. One of the best ways to measure the quality of oil by taste. The degree of bitterness is a close approximation of the level of lipid peroxides.

Your best source of high quality flaxseed oil will be found in health food stores. Most will offer several manufacturers to choose from. In general, most health food store brands are produced by special expeller extractions at temperatures below 6 degrees F, taking special care to protect the delicate oil from the damaging effects of heat, light, and oxygen.

Dr. Michael Murray notes the following guidelines for selecting a good flaxseed oil:

- Make sure flaxseed oil is derived from 100 percent third-party certified organic flaxseed. Oil expressed from non-organic flaxseed may contain pesticides and herbicides.
- Do not take the oil in capsule form. Your only assurance of quality is taste. Buy the oil in liquid form in opaque plastic bottles.
- Make sure the oil is as fresh as possible and not past the expiration date.
- Make sure that is clearly indicated that the oil is expeller-pressed.
- Use flaxseed oil high in lignans to gain the most benefit.

Additional Roles of Flaxseed Oil

We've so far discussed some impressive conclusions about the health benefits of flaxseed oil. But it appears that studies have only covered the tip of the iceberg. Because flaxseed research is in its infancy, it is likely that more uses will be uncovered in the future. Below is a summary of some uses for which flax is beginning to be recognized as useful therapy:

Allergies: Omega-3 oils may help to decrease allergic response.

Asthma: Flaxseed oil may noticeably relieve asthma within a few days after use.

Constipation: Eating flaxseed each day (baked into muffins or sprinkled on top of cereal of fruit) can increase the frequency of bowel movements.

Diabetes: The omega-3 oils in flaxseed oil have been shown to lower insulin requirements. Close monitoring is necessary. Flaxseed oil can also aid in circulation, which is an important factor in diabetes.

Inflammatory Conditions: Flaxseed oil likely will help to relieve the following inflammatory tissue conditions: water retention visual function, adrenal function, sperm formation.

PMS: Many forms of PMS can be relived within one month of using flax oil. Vitamins and herbs also contribute to control of premenstrual syndrome.

Recent Research

Results of recent studies indicate that consumption of Omega-3 fatty acids can benefit people women experiencing bone density loss, particularly in association with the onset of menopause. Researchers found that dietary supplementation with flaxseed oil reduces the production of cytokines—natural inflammatory produced in an aging woman's body. Some anti-inflammatory pharmaceuticals inhibit the production of cytokines (and eicosanoids), but flaxseed oil is a natural alternative. Evidence also points to the possible benefit of gamma-linolenic acid in preserving bone density.

In 2005, clinical investigations also suggested that EFAs also play an important role for normal function during growth and development and in the mediation of chronic disease. Thus, infants and pregnant and lactating women will benefit from including them in their diets. Researchers claim that once cardiovascular disease, hypertension, and autoimmune, allergic, and neurological disorders appear to respond to fatty acid supplementation, a diet balanced with these acids will decrease or delay their manifestation.

Conclusion

Because of its high omega-3 fatty acid content in the form of alpha-linolenic oil, flax packs great health benefits. Besides being an agent in the prevention of heart disease and conditions associated with it, flaxseed oil can help to improve skin problems and autoimmune disorders. Perhaps its greatest value lies in it ability to fight cancer due to its abundance of lignans. The omega-3 fatty acids in flaxseed oil are recommended for everyone because these essential nutrients are lacking in North American diets. Flaxseed oil supplementation can help your body function in the way that it was meant to.

References

Aldercreutz, H. Scandinavian Journal of clinical Laboratory Investigation, vol 50 (Suppl 201), (1992); 3-23.

Burr, G.O., and Burr, M.M. "A New Deficiency Disease Produced by the Rigid Exclusion of Fat From the Diet." The Journal of Biology and Chemistry, 82a (1929); 345-367

Chan, J.K., McDonale. B.E., Gerreard, J.M., bruce, V.M., Weaver, B.K., and Holub, B.J. "Effect of Dietary Alpha-linolenic Acid and Its Ratio to Linolenic Acid on Platelet and Plasma Fatty Acids and Thrombogenesis." Lipids, vol. 28 (1993); 811-817

Cnnane, S.C. et al. British Journal of Nutrition, vol. 69 (1993); 443-453

Ddyken, M.L., Wolf, P.A., Barnett, H.J.M., Bergan, J.J., Hass, W.K., Kannel, W.B., Kuller, L. Kurtzke, J.F., and Sundte T.M. "Risk Factors in Stroke: A statement for Physicians by the Subcommittee on Risk Factors and Stroke of the Stroke Council." Stroke, vol. 15 (1989); 1105-1111

Flax Council of Canada. http: www.flaxcouncil.ca/flaxnut5.html

Hartop P.J., and Prottey, C. "Changes in Transepidermal Water Loss and the Composition of Epidermal Lecithin After Applications of Pure Fatty Acid Triglycerides to the Skin of Essential Fatty Acid Deficient Rats." British Journal of Dermatology, vol. 95 (1976); 255-26

Kettler D. Alternative Medicine Review, 6: 61, 2004.

Manson, J.E., Tosteson, H., Ridker, P.M., Satterfield, S., Herbert, P., O'Connor, G.T., Buring, J.E., and Hennekens, C.H. "The Primary Prevention of Myocardial Infarction." New England Journal of Medicine 326 (1992); 1406-1416

Mercola, J., M.D. "Preventive Environmental Medicine." http://alt.medmarket.com/members.reidds/herbplus/info/herb3art.html

Mercola, J., M.D. "Preventive Environmental Medicine." http://alt.medmarket.com/members.reidds/herbplus/info/herb3art.html

Michnovica, Jon J. How to Reduce You Risk of Breast Cancer. New Yourk, NY: Warner Brooks, 1994; 54

Murray, Michael, N.D. Health Counselor Magazine. http://www.run-ti.com/mall/barleans/pages/flaxfacts/omega3.html

National Research Council. Diet and Health: Implications for Reducing Chronic Disease Risk. Washington, D.C.: National Academy Press, 1989:413-430, 549-561.

Nelson, G.J., and Chamberlain, J.G., In Flaxseed in Human Nutrition. Cunnane, S.C. and Thompson, L.U. eds., Champaign, Ill: AOCS Press, 1995: 187-206

Nettleton, J.A., "Omega-3 Fatty Acids: Comparison of Plant and Seafood Sources in Human Nutrition." Journal of the American Dietetics Association, vol. 91 (1991); 331-337

Nettleton, J.A., Omega-3 Fatty Acids and Health, New York, NY: Chapman and Hall, 1995: 34-35.

Oster G., and Thompson, D. Journal of American Dietetics Association, vol. 96

(1996); 127-131

Schmidt E.B. et al. "Proceedings from the Scientific Conference on Omega-3 Fatty Acids in Nutrition." Vascular Biology, and Medicine. Dallas, TX: American Heart Association, 1995: 208-213

Serrainoff and Thompson, L. Cancer Letters, 60 (1991); 135-142

Simopoulos A., Lipids, 34, Suppl 2005

Sinclair, H.M.. "Deficiency of Essentail Fatty Acids and Athersclerosis, etcetera." Lancet, I, (1956); 381-383.

Swank, R.L.. "Multiple Sclerosis. A Correlation of Its Incidence with Dietary Fat." American Journal of Medical Science, 220 (1950); 421-430.

Tate, G., Mandell B.F., Laposata, M., Ohliger, D., Baker, D.G., Schumacher, H.R., and Zurier R.B., "Suppression of Acute and Chronic Infalmmation by Dietary Gamma Linolenic Acid." Journal of Rheumatology, vol 16 (1989); 729

Ziboh, V.A., Cohen, K.A., Ellis, C.N., Miller, C., Hamilton, T., Kargballe, K., Hydrick, C.R., and Vorhees, J.J. "Effects of Dietary Supplementation of Fish Oil on Neutrophil and Epidermal Fatty Acids: Modulation of the Clinical Course of Psoratic Subjects." Archives of Dermatology, vol 122 (1986); 1277-1281.